MEDITERRANEAN DIET FOR OSTEOARTHRITIS

Stay Free From Osteoarthritis With The New And Tested Mediterranean Diet And Cook Plan For Beginners

Armstrong O. Mabel

Table of Contents

Chapter 1 3
   INTRODUCTION 3
   SYMPTOMS OF OSTEOARTHRITIS 4

Chapter 2 7
   WHAT IS OSTEOARTHRITIS 7
   CAUSES OF OSTEOARTHRITIS 10

Chapter 3 12
   RISK FACTORS 12
   IMPORTANT FACTS YOU SHOULD KNOW 14
   OSTEOARTHRITIS VERSUS ATROPHIC JOINT INFLAMMATION 16
   WHAT IS THE MEDITERRANEAN DIET? 18

Chapter 4 20
   MEDITERRANEAN DIET AND OSTEOARTHRITIS 20
   HOW IT WORK 21
   MEDITERRANEAN FOOD FOR OSTEOARTHRITIS 23

THE END 30

Chapter 1

INTRODUCTION

Osteoarthritis is that the commonest kind of joint pain, influencing numerous individuals around the world. It happens when the defensive ligament that pads the closures of your bones wears out over the long run.

In spite of the fact that osteoarthritis can harm any joint, the problem most commonly influences joints in your grasp, knees, hips and spine.

Osteoarthritis side effects can normally be overseen, albeit the harm to joints can't be switched.

Remaining dynamic, keeping a sound weight and a couple of medicines may moderate movement of the sickness and help improve torment and joint capacity.

SYMPTOMS OF OSTEOARTHRITIS

Osteoarthritis indications regularly grow gradually and deteriorate over the long run. Signs and manifestations of osteoarthritis include:

* Pain: Influenced joints may sting during or after development.

* Stiffness: Joint firmness could be generally observable after

arousing or subsequent to being idle.

* Tenderness: Your joint may feel delicate once you apply light strain to or close to it.

* Loss of adaptability: you would perhaps not be prepared to move your joint through its full scope of movement.

* Grating sensation: you would conceivably feel a grinding sensation once you utilize the joint, and you would potentially hear popping or snapping.

* Bone spikes: These additional pieces of bone, which want hard

bumps, can shape round the influenced joint.

* Swelling: This could be brought about by delicate tissue aggravation round the joint

Chapter 2

WHAT IS OSTEOARTHRITIS

Osteoarthritis might be a reformist condition with five phases, from 0 to 4. The essential stage (0) addresses a conventional joint. Stage 4 addresses serious Osteoarthritis. Not every person who has Osteoarthritis will advance all the gratitude to organize 4. The condition regularly balances out well before arriving at this stage.

Individuals with serious Osteoarthritis have broad or complete loss of ligament in at least one joint. The bone on bone grinding identified with this will cause serious manifestations, for example, increased growing and irritation. The amount of synovia inside the joint may increment. Regularly, this liquid lessens grinding during development. Nonetheless, in bigger sums, it can cause joint growing. Pieces of severed ligament can likewise glide inside the synovia, expanding agony and growing.

* Increased torment: you'll feel torment during exercises, yet in addition when you're very still. You'll sympathize with an ascent in your agony level on the grounds that the day advances, or more expanding in your joints in the

event that you've utilized them tons for the duration of the day.

* Decreased scope of movement. You'll not be prepared to move additionally, because of solidness or agony in your joints. This will make it harder to appreciate the everyday exercises that won't to come without any problem.

* Joint unsteadiness. Your joints may die down stable. For instance, on the off chance that you have extreme Osteoarthritis in your knees, you'll experience locking (abrupt absence of development). You'll additionally encounter clasping (when your knee gives

out), which may cause falls and injury.

* Other indications: As a joint keeps on influencing, muscle shortcoming, bone prods, and joint disfigurement can likewise happen.

CAUSES OF OSTEOARTHRITIS

Osteoarthritis happens when the ligament that pads the closures of bones in your joints step by step crumbles. Ligament might be a firm, dangerous tissue that grants almost frictionless joint movement. In the end, if the ligament wears out totally, bone will rub on bone.

Osteoarthritis has regularly been referenced as a "mileage" sickness. However, other than the breakdown of ligament, osteoarthritis influences the entire joint. It causes changes inside the bone and decay of the connective tissues that hold the joint together and affix muscle to bone. It likewise causes irritation of the joint covering.

Chapter 3

RISK FACTORS

Components which will build your danger of osteoarthritis include:

* Older age: the threat of osteoarthritis increments with age.

: Sex: Ladies are bound to create osteoarthritis, however it isn't clear why.

* Obesity: Conveying additional weight adds to osteoarthritis severally, and subsequently the more you gauge, the more noteworthy your danger. Expanded weight adds pressure to weight-bearing joints, similar to your hips and knees. Likewise, fat

tissue produces proteins which will cause unsafe irritation in and around your joints.

* Joint wounds: Wounds, similar to individuals who happen when playing sports or from a mishap, can expand the threat of osteoarthritis. Indeed, even wounds that happened a couple of year's prior and apparently recuperated can expand your danger of osteoarthritis.

* Repeated weight on the joint: In the event that your work or a game you play places redundant weight on a joint, that joint may in the long run create osteoarthritis.

* Bone distortions: Some persons are brought into the world with deformed joints or faulty ligament.

* Certain metabolic sicknesses: These incorporate diabetes and a condition during which your body has an extreme measure of iron.

IMPORTANT FACTS YOU SHOULD KNOW

Osteoarthritis might be a condition that deteriorates after some time, regularly prompting persistent agony. Joint torment and solidness can get sufficiently serious to frame day by day assignments troublesome.

Sorrow and rest aggravations may result from the torment and handicap of osteoarthritis.

* Osteoarthritis and ligament: Ligament might be an extreme, rubbery substance that is adaptable and milder than bone. Its responsibility is to watch the finishes of bones inside a joint and grant them to move effectively against each other. At the point when ligament separates, these bone surfaces become hollowed and unpleasant. This will cause torment inside the joint, and aggravation in encompassing tissues. Harmed ligament can't fix itself. This is regularly on the

grounds that ligament doesn't contain any veins.

At the point when ligament erodes totally, the padding cushion that it gives vanishes, permitting bone-on-bone contact. This will cause exceptional torment and different indications identified with Osteoarthritis.

OSTEOARTHRITIS VERSUS ATROPHIC JOINT INFLAMMATION

Osteoarthritis and atrophic joint inflammation share an identical side effect however are totally different conditions. Osteoarthritis might be a degenerative condition, which proposes that it expansions in seriousness after some time. Atrophic joint inflammation, on the contrary hand, is an immune system infection.

Individuals with atrophic joint inflammation have invulnerable frameworks that botch the delicate coating around joints to be a danger to the body, making it assault that zone. This delicate coating, which consolidates the synovia, is named the synovium. Since the framework dispatches its attack, liquid development inside the joint happens, causing solidness, torment, growing, and aggravation.

WHAT IS THE MEDITERRANEAN DIET?

The eating regimen stresses privately developed foods grown from the ground, sound fats like vegetable oil and nuts, entire grains and a couple of fish, yogurt and wine . It's the path individuals in Greece and southern Italy have eaten for many years, and it's credited for their long lives and low paces of diabetes, heftiness, heart condition and dementia. The sickness battling force of the Mediterranean eating routine stems from its capacity to oversee irritation by that represent considerable authority in calming food sources (berries, fish, olive oil) and barring or restricting favorable to incendiary ones (red meat, sugar and most dairy). Osteoarthritis is currently known to have an incendiary segment, so this way of eating can cause genuine upgrades in joint agony

Chapter 4

MEDITERRANEAN DIET AND OSTEOARTHRITIS

If an equilibrium diet, shifted and sound impacts decidedly in our wellbeing and diminishes the threat of the numerous infections.

It is known since a brief timeframe that Mediterranean Diet includes an ideal impact on cardiovascular wellbeing, a few kinds of malignant growth, ongoing illnesses and psychological productivity; could be useful for joint wellbeing and osteoarthritis.

The part of sustenance in persistent pathologies is by and

large more contemplated and accordingly the example of the Mediterranean Diet has been related with the decrease of knee aggravation in patients with atrophic joint pain, this is frequently the reasoning why the impact that would wear osteoarthritis was examined, also

HOW IT WORK

Mediterranean Diet secures and helps in osteoarthritis severally:

* It favors the norm of lifetime of individuals with osteoarthritis by diminishing irritation, improving the scope of joints development and improving their state of mind.

* it's a defensive impact of the osteoarthritis, on account of individuals that best follow the Mediterranean Diet have less instances of osteoarthritis (that is to make reference, to the predominance of osteoarthritis is lower).

* It goes about as a mitigating diet, as a result of the parts present in specific food varieties normal for this food design that have the property of decreasing the provocative substance and accordingly the corruption of the ligament.

MEDITERRANEAN FOOD FOR OSTEOARTHRITIS

Counting explicit food sources inside the eating routine can fortify the bones, muscles, and joints and assist the body with battling aggravation and infection.

Individuals with osteoarthritis can have a go at adding the ensuing eight food sources to their eating routine to facilitate their manifestations:

* Sleek fish: Salmon contains numerous omega-3 unsaturated fats, which have mitigating properties.

Slick fish contain numerous stimulating omega-3 unsaturated fats. These polyunsaturated fats have calming properties all together that they may profit individuals with osteoarthritis.

Individuals with osteoarthritis should intend to disintegrate least one part of slick fish each week. Sleek fish include:

a. sardines

b. mackerel

c. salmon

d. new fish

The individuals who like to not eat fish can take supplements that contain omega-3 all things considered, similar to creature oil, krill oil, or linseed oil.

Different wellsprings of omega-3 incorporate chia seeds, linseed oil, and pecans. These food sources likewise can assist with battling aggravation.

* Oils: Notwithstanding slick fish, oil can lessen irritation. Additional virgin vegetable oil contains undeniable degrees of oleocanthal, which can have comparative properties to nonsteroidal mitigating drug drugs. Avocado

and safflower oils are stimulating choices and ought to likewise assist with bringing down cholesterol.

* Dairy: Milk, yogurt, and cheddar are plentiful in calcium and nutrient D. These supplements increment bone strength, which can improve excruciating manifestations. Dairy additionally contains proteins which will assist with making muscle. Individuals that are having the opportunity to deal with their weight can pick low-fat choices.

* Dull verdant greens: Dull verdant greens are plentiful in

nutrient D and stress-battling phytochemicals and cell reinforcements. Nutrient D is significant for calcium assimilation and may likewise support the framework, assisting the body with repulsing disease.

Dull verdant greens include:

a. spinach

b. kale

c. chard

d. collard greens

* Broccoli: Broccoli contains a compound called sulforaphane, which specialists accept could

moderate the movement of osteoarthritis. This vegetable is furthermore plentiful in nutrients K and C, likewise as bone-fortifying calcium.

* Green tea: Polyphenols are cell reinforcements that specialists accept could likewise be prepared to decrease irritation and moderate the speed of ligament harm. Tea contains undeniable degrees of polyphenols.

* Garlic: A compound called diallyl disulfide that occurs in garlic may conflict with the chemicals inside the body that harm ligament.

* Nuts: Nuts are useful for the guts and contain undeniable degrees of calcium, magnesium, zinc, nutrient E, and fiber. They additionally contain omega-3 unsaturated fat which helps the framework.

THE END

Made in the USA
Columbia, SC
24 January 2025